PURE
Beauty
NATURALLY

Linda Lee

Balboa Press books may be ordered through booksellers or by contacting:

Balboa Press
A Division of Hay House
1663 Liberty Drive
Bloomington, IN 47403
www.balboapress.com
1 (877) 407-4847

ISBN: 978-1-5043-6180-4 (sc)
ISBN: 978-1-5043-6179-8 (e)

Print information available on the last page.

Balboa Press rev. date: 10/14/2016

BALBOA.
PRESS
A DIVISION OF HAY HOUSE

Contents

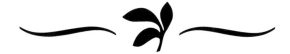

This book is dedicated to my daughters Tracy and Sheri

and my granddaughters Natalee and Ellianna.

May you always remember your true essence and beauty

and honor the divine feminine within …

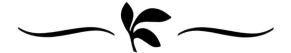

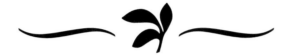

SECTION ONE

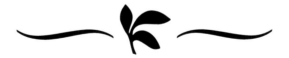

Lemongrass

There is a special place in my heart for Lemongrass. My earliest recollection
of anyone drinking tea is my Grandmother Ida who drank this sweet-smelling
tea. I love it to this day for so many reasons, including its taste, smell and ability
to do amazing things for the body and mind. I simply love the smell!

Lemongrass is used on many levels for purification.

It supports digestion, the lymphatic system and promotes higher levels of awareness.

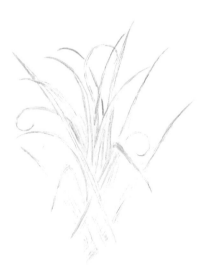

A Bit About Ingredients

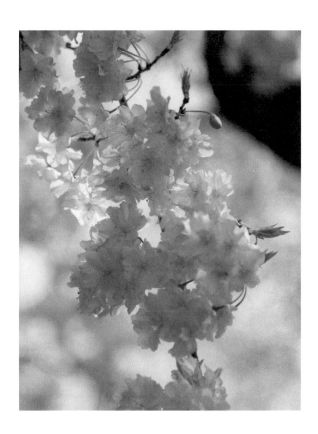

Coconut and Jojoba Oils*: Natural sunscreens, many healing attributes as well.

Vegetable Glycerin: Attracts moisture if water present, dries skin if not.

Therapeutic Grade Essential Oils*: Their chemical makeup has been preserved, powerful healing agents, absorbs easily and efficiently.

Cold-Pressed Oils: No heat has been applied which preserves their chemical makeup therefore all nutrients therein.

Witch Hazel: This protects the skin, soothes it, and is an amazing skin healer which will enhance the effects of the amazing oils you will combine with it.

See Resource Page

Lavender

Lavender is a beloved oil to many. It's an all around oil that has so many uses beyond just its calming effects on the mind or for burns. It has the ability to regenerate tissue. It's also used for cleansing and soothing to the skin. It can be used for a wide variety of skin conditions, used as an aid for hair loss, and more. It can also help improve mental accuracy and concentration. This is an oil that everyone needs to have on hand!

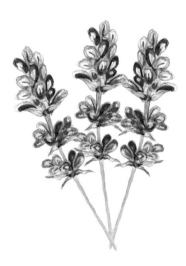

Why These Recipes were Created

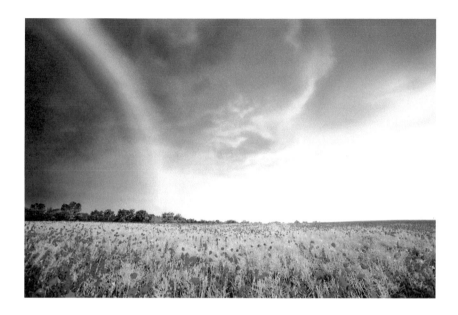

All of the recipes in this booklet were created from necessity and definitely labors of love for my body and now yours! They were a necessity in the sense that I could not find quality products without alcohol, Sodium Lauryl Sulfate (SLS), propyl glycols, petroleum products and other harmful ingredients.

I will admit I have become a bit of a purist when it comes to what I put on my body. Not too long ago I was watching a program on television that talked about hair, and they suggested that it doesn't matter what you put on your hair 'it's dead'. While this may be true, the skin and pores the hair attaches to are not dead, and we are still absorbing into our systems all we put onto our head and even what we put on our nails.

My first creation were the lip balms. Many years ago I found a lip balm that had a beautiful consistency and to my knowledge at the time the ingredients were good. As happens often in life I could no longer find that product after a couple of years.

I took a class more than 20 years ago to learn to make lip balms. I was a bit horrified to see the instructor using cake flavoring for flavors, hydrogenated cooking oil for the base, and a microwave to heat the ingredients. As with all recipes however her recipe was simply a guide. I then had the basics on how to make them, and I was off and running.

I began making my own skin toner as well. There was a very popular brand I used back in the 1970's and 80's. As I became more aware I realized that the alcohol used, most likely for preserving the toner, was actually drying my skin. When using pure, high quality, therapeutic-grade essential oils as ingredients, preservatives are not necessary!

The floral sprays originated from a desire to have a quick refresher that was safe to spray on my face and around my eyes (not in the eyes). The first one I ever experienced was orange, and I fell in love with these little luxuries I keep around the house and my office now.

Hair rinse, let's face it, this was pure and simple to save money! The hair conditioners on the market that do not have sulphates or petroleum products are few and far between if you can find them at all, and if you can find them they are expensive. My recipe is so simple and my hair feels just as good if not better using this simple rinse. You will find those and more in this little book.

The point is to all of this is to begin with what we put on our body to clean up pollution! Our inner environment affects our outer environment. If you've ever walked by someone and whatever they are wearing literally gets stuck in your nose or throat you know what I mean.

Be the Goddess you are meant to be! Purify your life, improve your emotions and love yourself enough to give yourself the best!

Melissa

Sweet Melissa …

Since ancient times, this oil has been used for nervous
disorders and ailments of the heart and emotions.

It's also helpful for depression, anxiety and insomnia.

It has the ability of calming yet uplifting the spirit and also balancing the emotions. It
assists in removing emotional blocks and brings about a positive outlook on life.

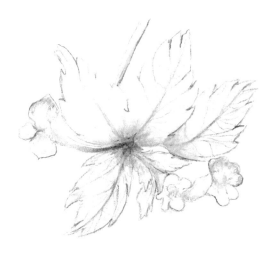

Be Aware!

Be as aware of what you put ON your body as what you put IN to your body. It only takes 26 seconds for chemicals in your personal care products to enter your blood stream!

What's in your shampoo, eye shadow, body lotion, hair styling products, foundation, blusher, lipstick, deodorant, fake tanning products, foundation, nail polish or remover, perfume, mouthwash or toothpaste? There could be an average of 475 chemicals in these products, and the biggest culprit is synthetic perfumes that contain approximately 250 chemicals!

It's time for you to love yourself enough to surround yourself with the best life has to offer! You will also give yourself the gift of emotional, mental and physical wellbeing that has no price tag.

THE RECIPES

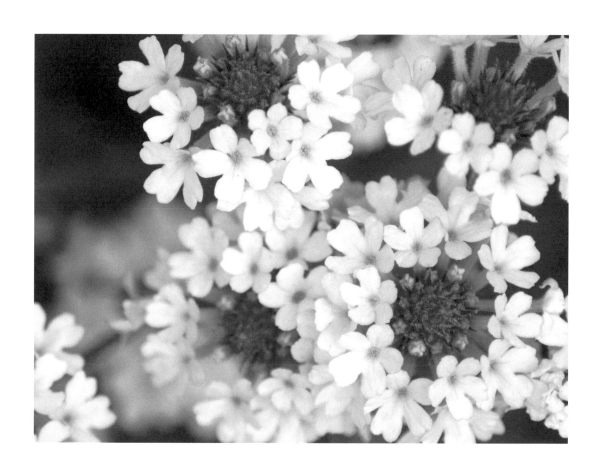

Lip Balm

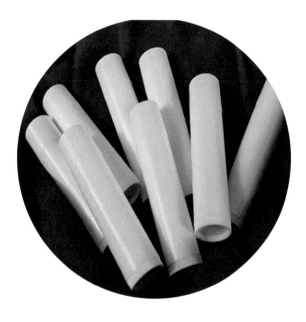

2 oz. of oil ~ a combination of

cold-pressed coconut, olive (ratio is 45/45% each) and Jojoba oil (10%)

1 oz. unfiltered bees wax

**3 oz. makes 15 roll-up tubes

Melt these ingredients together. I use a Pyrex measuring cup putting the handle over the side of a saucepan of boiling water (double-boiler concept). I use wood skewers to stir.**

Then add several drops of Vitamin E Oil, Calendula Extract and 60-90 drops of Essential Oil* (optional).

**Test one balm pouring it into a container and let set before pouring them all so adjustments to the texture can be made to personal desire.*

I love orange Essential Oil, however you can use lavender, grapefruit, citrus oils or whatever you like!

Cedarwood

I love to be around Cedar trees, and this oil keeps me
connected to the power and beauty of these trees.

Cedarwood stimulates the brain's limbic region (the center of our emotions) and the Pineal
Gland which releases Melatonin. It's also calming, purifying, and is heavenly to smell …

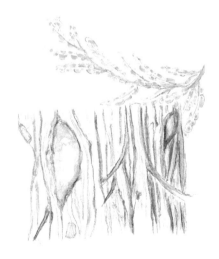

Skin Toners

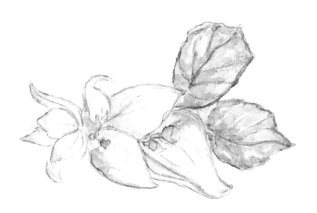

4 oz. squeeze bottle ~

*Pour in approximately 2/3 to 3/4 oz. of vegetable glycerin

The glycerin will help glide the oil/water over the face – too sticky, too much, not enough it will just feel like water – and it needs to stay on skin.

*Fill the bottle with pure water

*Add your favorite Therapeutic Grade Essential Oils at 5 drops each. Three to Five different oils are ideal.

After cleansing your skin, gently shake the bottle back and forth a few times and apply to your face with a cotton ball.

My favorites are Geranium, Lavender, Rosewood, Frankincense, Ylang Ylang, Lemongrass, Patchouli and Sandalwood.

**Customize for your skins needs!

Sandalwood

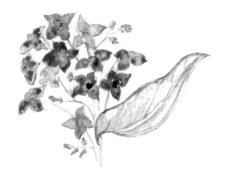

One of my very favorites.

Sandalwood has amazing healing properties and supports and stimulates the immune system.

It enhances deep sleep, helps to remove negative programming at the cellular level. It's high in sesquiterpenes that stimulate the pineal and limbic region of the brain and a powerful healer, and it's grounding and stabilizing.

Floral Water

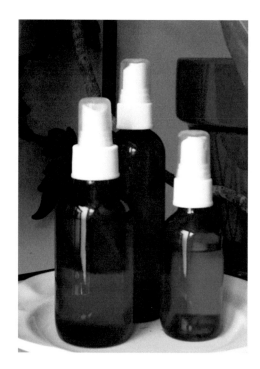

These are easy, easy …

4 oz. sprayer bottle

Fill with 6.0 acidic water (perfect balance for skin) or pure, clean water.

Add 9 drops (depending on preference) of your favorite Therapeutic Grade Essential Oils.

*** You can use these on your face (avoid eye contact), your body, as air refresher or on bedding (will not stain).

Frankincense

The King of Oils and considered the "Holy Anointing Oil"!

Used to treat every conceivable ill known to man and valued more than gold in ancient times.

Very high in sesquiterpenes and affects the limbic region of the brain
and hypothalamus, which is considered the master gland.

It's known to increase spiritual awareness, improve attitude, and uplift your spirit.

Worth its weight in gold …

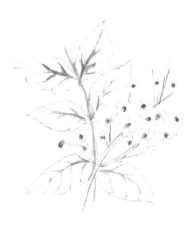

Yoga Mat Cleaner

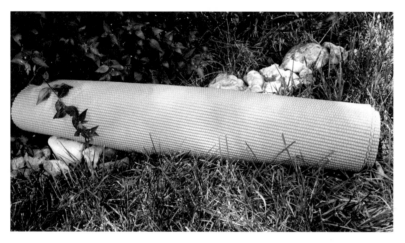

4 oz. spray bottle 1 oz. each of ~

*Dr. Bronner's Unscented Castile Soap

* White Vinegar

3 oz. of Pure Clean Water

Therapeutic Grade Essential Oils ~

6 drops each of Tea Tree and Lemon Oil

Wipe down both sides of your mat with the cleaner and then wipe down a second time with a fresh, clean, damp cloth.

TIP: Instead of rolling your mat, fold it. This way you don't roll the floor side of your mat onto the side that you practice your sacred yoga on.

Jasmine

Can't you smell it now...

Women treasure Jasmine for its beautiful seductive fragrance.

It will help with depression, aging skin, and it's stimulating and uplifting.

It's lovely to have around you anytime.

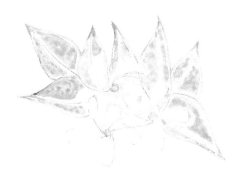

What is Samadhi?

The highest stage in meditation in which a person experiences oneness with the universe.

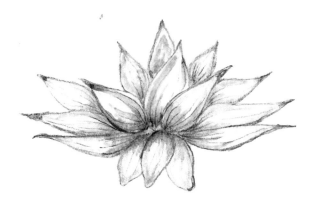

Samadhi

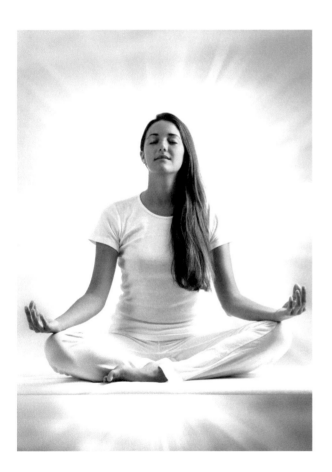

Spray ~

2 oz. spray bottle, filled with pure, clean water.

6 drops each of Frankincense and Rose Therapeutic Grade Essential Oils.

Will enhance your quiet, sacred spaces.

Spray on you and around you...

Oil ~

1/2 oz. beautiful perfume bottle filled with Jojoba Oil* and 3 drops each of Frankincense and Rose Oil.

Enhance your meditative experience by placing a drop or two at the space between your eyebrows, also known as the third-eye area.

* See Resource Page

Ylang Ylang

The flower of flowers!

Helps to regulate the heartbeat, just think all it can help around that!

Balances the female/male energies, enhances spiritual attunement, increases focus of thoughts, and filters negative energy. Restores confidence and peace.

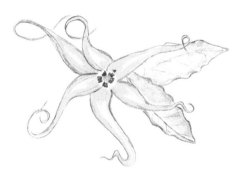

Massage Oils

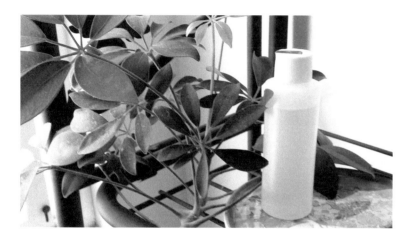

4 oz. squeeze bottle

Fill with cold-pressed Almond Oil

Add 25 drops of your favorite Therapeutic Grade Essential Oils for relaxation.

*Some of my favorites are Stress Away, Lavender, Mandarin, Orange, Lemongrass, Frankincense, Bergamont, Geranium, Eucalyptus Globulas and Sandalwood. Getting creative is half the fun!

Patchouli

Yes, many of us have certain ideas about this amazing oil.

However, once you get to know it you may use it every day of your life, as I do.

Aside from its many health properties such as a digestive aid and relaxant it also softens wrinkles, aids dry skin, and so much more. This beautiful oil helps to clarify thoughts, assisting in the release of unhealthy jealousy, obsessions and insecurities.

Belly Oil

For Moms-to-Be

2 oz. squeeze bottle

Add 1/4 oz. each of Avocado and Wheat Germ Oil

Add 3/4 oz. each of Cold-Pressed Sesame and Almond Oil

Here are some nice blends of Therapeutic Grade Essential Oils 3 drops each of ~

* Lavender, Rosewood and Geranium

* Lemon, Jasmine and Chamomile

* Bergamont, Ylang Ylang, Palmarosa and Rose

Rose

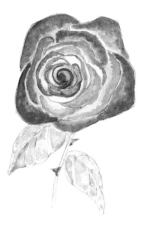

The Queen of Oils!

Used for thousands of years for anything you can think of for the skin.

Its beautiful fragrance is intoxicating and can act as an aphrodisiac.

It's emotionally balancing, elevates the mind, and creates a sense of well-being.

Insect Repellant

Therapeutic Grade Essential Oils ~

* Citronella   * Idaho Tansy
* Cedarwood   * Tea Tree
* Eucalyptus Citriodora   * Geranium

6 drops each of the oils in a 4 oz. spray bottle filled with Witch Hazel

* I love this spray when I'm hiking. It has NO chemicals, dirt won't stick to it, and it's highly effective!

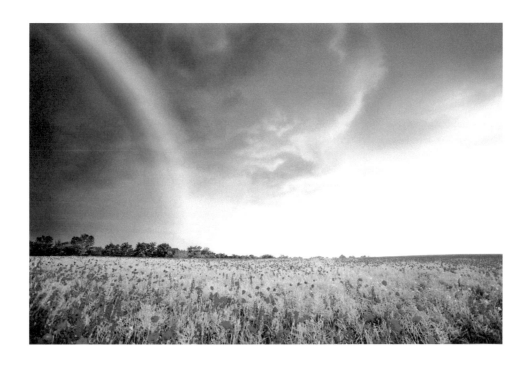

Geranium

I wear Geranium every day.

It heals and regenerates skin, improves blood flow, cleanses and revitalizes the skin.

It also helps to release negative memories and nervous tension by balancing the emotions, lifting your spirit, and bringing feelings of peace, well-being and hope.

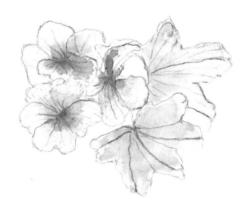

Simple Hair Rinse

1 - 16 oz. squeeze bottle

1 –Tbsp of Apple Cider Vinegar

1 – Drop of your favorite Essential Oil

Put ingredients in the bottle and when ready to use fill with water and rinse through your hair thoroughly, and then a final rinse with fresh water.

Essential Oils for your hair ~

Rosemary – For hair loss, adds body and conditions hair

Lavender – Cleansing, balances pH

Tea Tree – Dandruff

Sandalwood – Graying Hair

Rosewood – Lightens Hair

Rosemary

I love Rosemary. It's a delicate plant, and when it flowers it is so beautiful.
It's as strong as it is delicate. If you've ever gotten a good whiff of Rosemary
you know it will sharpen your mind right away, bringing clarity and focus.
When we're alert and present we become less anxious in life.

It was also one of the highly effective protecting herbs that was used during
the plague to protect the thieves of the day from contracting disease.

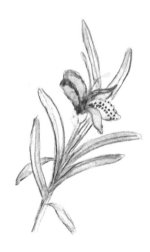

Oral Hygiene

How aware are you really about what you put in your mouth? We know about food, do we think about our mouthwash, toothpaste or tooth whiteners beyond what we're told they will do on the label or in the commercials? We should never use something for oral hygiene that we cannot swallow, as it's being absorbed into every part of your body in your mouth as you use it. You want to avoid products with laurel sodium sulphate, propyl glycols, aluminum, and the big one – fluoride.

Fluoride is simply a poison and affects every part of your body. We've been sold a bill of goods when it comes to fluoride – and not that I'm a big fan of the FDA but it's never been approved by them! We are told it strengthens tooth enamel and re-mineralizes the teeth to stop tooth decay. It's actually an aluminum waste byproduct. It was used during World War II to keep the prisoners docile. The definition of docile is *"ready to accept control or instruction; submissive."* I encourage you to educate yourself around this subject, it's important.

It's in everything, including your tooth whiteners. Some cities still put it in the water system (do you know where your bottled water comes from?), toothpaste, and if you want to double down get fluoride treatments at your dentist office! Children are most susceptible to this poison because as adults we're guilted into it or we just accept that the powers that be know what they're talking about — they're brainwashed too!!

Awareness, proper oral hygiene and thoughtful food intake can eradicate tooth decay! Unfortunately, we are a society that lives with little conscious thought, and we are easy prey for a cure-all after the fact to continue living without awareness of our health as we eat sugary, starchy, refined carbohydrates that are harmful to our teeth. These substances linger in your mouth, breaking down into simple sugars and creating bacteria that feeds on sugars that produce acid, which cause tooth decay.

Here are some reference sites to begin – http://fluoridealert.org/issues/health/facts/

https://www.organicconsumers.org/old_articles/body- care/toxic_cosmetics.php

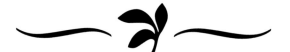

Simple Mouthwash

One drop* of Therapeutic Grade Essential Clove Oil to a slightly less than a mouth full of water. Swish and swallow, it's safe and you'll get added benefits!

* There are 300 drops to a 15 ml. bottle of oil. A bottle of Clove Oil will last almost one year, and it's safe to swallow. You would not think of swallowing a commercial-brand mouthwash ever!

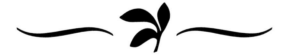

Clove

This versatile spice translates into a powerful healing Essential Oil.

This oil assists you in aging gracefully and assists in any type of infection you may have.

It's also a mental stimulant, assists in sleep, stimulates dreaming,
and creates a sense of protection and courage.

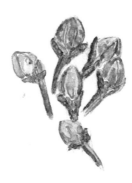

Oil Pulling

I've included this very important daily practice for several reasons. The benefits of this are many. Anything that you put into your mouth must be scrutinized. Each of our teeth are connected to different systems in the body, so if you're having a toothache you want to be aware of what's going on in the corresponding area of the body*.

Some of the benefits are it promotes whiter teeth, increases energy, detoxifies the body, helps to balance hormones, creates more beautiful skin, reduces or eliminates headaches, promotes oral hygiene, and more. This process literally pulls toxins out through the gums.

So Oil Pulling is easy and yet a bit time consuming. This is an Auyrvedic practice, and the oil traditionally used in this practice is organic, unrefined, cold-pressed Sesame Oil* or Coconut Oil* can also be used.

Put approximately 1 Tbsp of either oil in your mouth first thing in the morning before you do anything. Swish around in your mouth for 20 minutes. The oil will become watery, white and thin. Spit out and then brush your teeth.

Do this every morning and you'll begin to see amazing results. You'll get sick less often and feel and look great!

*Go to resources to find an amazing link to a chart, oils and article.

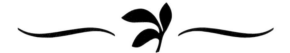

SECTION TWO

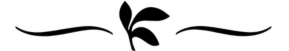

Sunscreens

Ok let's just look at the most common active ingredients in many sunscreens. The first one is Avobenzone which is a derivative of dibenzoylmethane which is a derivative of acetylacetone and then there's oxybenzone derived from the benzophenone group of chemicals. Chemicals being the key word.

As mentioned it only takes 26 seconds for our skin to absorb these and they are potentially harmful to you! Yes, they make them smell good and soak right into your skin easily (scary) yet we don't know the long term health risks.

Remember we need approximately 30 minutes of sunshine per day to produce the D3 Hormone, we also need it because it produces Serotonin (the feel good hormone) which in turns produces Melatonin to help us sleep at night. We have been sold a bill of goods, do your research and understand that Mother Nature has not made any mistakes, the Sun is not our enemy unless we believe it and then we find our self creating according to our thoughts!

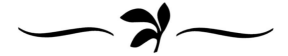

Natural Sunscreens

Raspberry Seed Oil	30 SPF
Wheat Germ Oil	20 SPF
Avocado Oil	15 SPF
Carrot Seed Oil**	10 SPF
Soy Oil	10 SPF
Coconut Oil**	8 SPF
Olive Oil	8 SPF
Macadamia Nut Oil	6 SPF
Almond Oil	5 SPF
Jojoba Oil**	4 SPF

* Remember to be responsible in the sun and also be aware that you need the sun for your health and well- being. The above oils when cold pressed, organic and unrefined will nourish and protect your skin at the same time without the unknown side effects of chemicals.

** See Resources Page.

What is an Essential Oil?

Knowing where the seeds come from first and foremost and caring where they come from. The seeds are organically grown, watered with clear, clean water that may even be infused with these life-giving oils, freshly cultivated so the plant is at its most optimal value, and then steam distilled with state of the art distillers to preserve the cellular structure and the delicate chemical compounds that make a plant extremely healing to your body — your temple of the mind and spirit; then respectfully and beautifully bottled so they are as treasured gifts on your shelf.

Essential Oils in Young Living's collection are life- enhancing gifts from the plant kingdom. Plants that have been revered for centuries for their beneficial and life-enhancing properties. Pure Essential Oils have re-emerged as a key solution to the challenges facing modern lifestyles without chemicals and dangerous side effects. Therapeutic Grade Essential Oils deliver support to the body through the skin, by smell and ingestion. Young Living is the only Company I trust as they have the highest standards for their farms and processing and exceed what the government standards are! These products are simply impeccable, of high integrity and come from a deep place of love created from the heart of Gary Young.

When love is infused with whatever you do, the vibration rises and the benefits exponentially change to a higher degree. Young Living's Essential Oils offer support to many systems of the mind, body and spirit. Because herbs and plants already have value for the human body when you have their "pure essence," there is the potential for amazing results naturally and without harmful side effects. This is the ultimate of what nature intended! Because these oils are energetically "pure essence," they work from not only a physical level, they also effect those intangible levels of emotions, mental and spiritual states. The benefits are many.

Thank you for coming along on this journey of discovery with me. You will begin to understand your pure essence when taking care and honoring yourself in a most beautiful way.

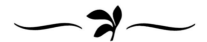

Our Amazing World of Natural Healing

From left to right:

Rosewood Tree, Citronella, Bergamot, Orange, Eucalyptus Tree, Mandarin,

Tea Tree, Chamomile, Lemon, Tansy, Palmarosa, Grapefruit

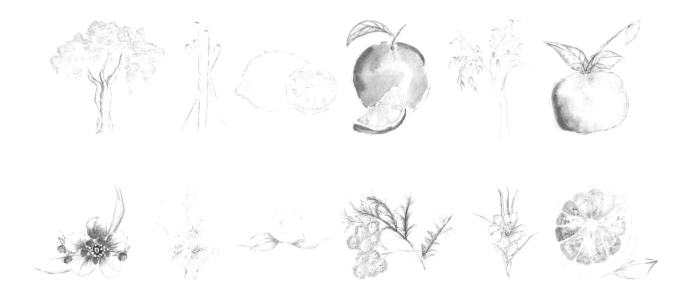

Essential Oil Benefits

Bergamot – Great for skin conditions, oily skin, mood lifting.

Cedarwood – A variety of skin conditions, hair loss.

Citrus Fresh – A nice blend of all the citruses.

Citronella – For healthy glowing skin; its lemony smell deflects insects.

Clove – Tooth pain, reduces bacteria and supports the immune system.

Eucalyptus Citriodora – Insect repellent.

Eucalyptus Globulus – Insect repellent, soothes sore muscles, purification.

Frankincense – Amazing healing oil and lifts spirits.

Geranium – Regenerates, healing to the skin, improves blood, cleansing, detoxifying, revitalizing.

Grapefruit – Detoxifying, refreshing (avoid applying to skin that will be exposed to sunlight).

Idaho Tansy – Insect repellent, skin conditions, tones entire system.

Jasmine – Skin conditions, a most beautiful fragrance that lifts the spirit of all around her.

Lavender – Healing to the skin, cleansing, calming.

Resources

Jojoba Oil

http://www.laronnajojoba.com/

Coconut Oil

http://healingtherapiesplacerville.com/health-benefits- of-coconut-oil/

Sesame Oil

http://healingtherapiesplacerville.com/links/

Become a member of Young Living for the highest quality Essential Oils

http://healingtherapiesplacerville.com/links/youngliving-essential-oils-2/

Continue your education of Essential Oils with the Essential Oil Desk Reference

https://www.discoverlsp.com/

Chart of teeth and their connection to the parts of the body

http://naturaldentistry.us/holistic-dentistry/meridian- tooth-chart-from-encinitas-dentist/

Article on Oil Pulling

http://healingtherapiesplacerville.com/939-2/

About the Author

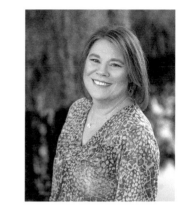

Linda Lee has been in the Holistic Field for more than 35 years. She is a Holistic Health Expert Specializing in Clinical Hypnotherapy, and Internationally published author and speaker.

Linda is so happy to bring her personal recipes to you! This is a gift from her heart and something she wanted to get out into the world.

In its simplicity, she wanted you to know how you can care for yourself naturally without chemicals, easily made at home, with the highest quality of ingredients including love, giving you peace of mind that what you are introducing to your body is not only safe, additionally you are gaining amazing positive side benefits.

These days it is so important to get back to basics and say no to what is harming your body, mind, spirit and our planet – taking responsibility and educating yourself is key.

Go to her website for more information at www.discoveryourpower.net.

Printed in the United States
By Bookmasters